800 Calorie Diet Cookbook For Weight-loss

Recipes for a Healthy Lifestyle

Published by Crown Publishers

Contents

Understanding Weight Loss

Losing weight can seem like a daunting task. But with a few simple tips, you can get on the path towards a healthier, happier you. Understanding the basics of weight loss can help you create an effective plan to reach your goals. The first step in understanding weight loss is recognizing the importance of nutrition. Eating a balanced diet with plenty of fruits and vegetables, lean proteins, and healthy grains can help you shed pounds. You should also limit your intake of processed foods, sugary snacks, and unhealthy fats. Staying hydrated and getting plenty of rest can also help with weight loss. The next step is understanding how physical activity plays a role in weight loss. Exercise helps to burn calories and build muscle, both of which can help you lose weight. Try to incorporate a variety of activities into your weight loss plan, and be sure to set achievable goals so you don't become frustrated. Finally, understanding the psychological aspects of weight loss is essential. Developing a positive attitude and focusing on your goals can help you stay motivated and make healthier choices. Seeking professional help can also be beneficial if you're having a hard time sticking to your weight loss plan. Understanding weight loss can be the key to successfully reaching your goals. With the right nutrition, physical activity, and psychological approach, you can take control of your health and achieve the body you've always wanted.

Trying to lose weight can be an overwhelming process. But by understanding the basics of weight loss, you can develop a plan that works for you. The first step in understanding weight loss is recognizing the importance of nutrition. Eating a balanced diet full of fruits, vegetables, and lean proteins is essential for weight loss. Try to limit your intake of processed foods, sugary snacks, and unhealthy fats. Hydration and adequate rest are also important. The next step is understanding the role of physical activity in weight loss. Exercise helps to burn calories and build muscle, which is key to losing weight. Aim to incorporate a variety of activities into your plan, and be sure to set realistic goals. Finally, understanding the psychological aspects of weight loss is critical. Developing a positive attitude and focusing on your goals can help keep you motivated and make healthier choices. If you're having a hard time, consider seeking professional help. Weight loss doesn't have to be a difficult process. By understanding the basics and creating an effective plan, you can take control of your health and reach your goals. With determination and consistency, you can achieve the body you've always wanted.

What Causes Weight Gain?

Weight gain is a complex problem that can have a variety of causes, from hormonal imbalances to poor dietary habits. Although weight gain can be a symptom of certain medical conditions, it often occurs when a person consumes more calories than their body is able to burn off. In this article, we will explore some of the common causes of weight gain and how to address them.

Hormonal Imbalances: Hormonal imbalances can be caused by a variety of factors, including stress, a poor diet, and lack of sleep. Imbalances in hormones such as insulin, thyroid hormones, and cortisol can lead to an increase in appetite and fat storage, resulting in weight gain. If you suspect that a hormonal imbalance may be causing your weight gain, speak to your doctor to discuss potential treatments.

Poor Diet: Eating too many calories, especially from unhealthy sources such as highly processed foods, can lead to weight gain. Consuming too many calories can also lead to insulin resistance, which in turn can cause further weight gain. To prevent weight gain, focus on eating a balanced diet, limiting processed foods, and eating plenty of fresh fruits and vegetables.

Lack of Exercise: Exercise helps to burn off excess calories and can also help to regulate hormone levels. People who don't get enough exercise are more likely to gain weight, as the extra calories they consume are not being burned off. To prevent weight gain, aim for at least 30 minutes of physical activity a day.

Genetics: Genetics can play a role in weight gain, as certain genes may make a person more likely to gain weight. If you have a family history of obesity, it is important to take extra measures to ensure you maintain a healthy weight.

Medications: Certain medications, such as steroids, can cause weight gain. If you have recently started a new medication and have noticed an increase in weight, it is important to speak to your doctor to discuss alternative medications or other solutions.

Emotional Eating: Eating in response to emotions, such as boredom, stress, or sadness, can lead to weight gain. If you find yourself emotionally eating, it is important to try to address the underlying cause of the emotion and to find healthier ways to cope.

Age: As you age, your body's metabolism slows down, resulting in a decrease in the number of calories you burn. This can lead to weight gain if you don't make changes to your lifestyle, such as reducing your calorie intake and increasing your physical activity.

Overall, weight gain can be caused by a variety of factors, including hormonal imbalances, poor diet, lack of exercise, genetics, medications, and emotional eating. If you think you may be gaining weight because of any of these factors, it is important to speak to your doctor to discuss potential solutions.

Very Low-Calorie Diets: What You Need to Know

When you're on a low-calorie diet, you usually get between 800 and 1,500 calories a day. For some people, an alternative for short-term weight loss is a very low-calorie diet.

Many very low-calorie diets are commercially-made formulas of 800 calories or fewer that replace all the food you usually eat. Others, such as the well-known grapefruit diet rely on eating a lot of the same low-calorie food or foods.

Very low-calorie diets are not the same as over-the-counter meal replacements, which you substitute for one or two meals a day.

How Effective Are Very Low-Calorie Diets?

If you have a BMI over 30 (which your doctor will call "obese"), then a very low-calorie diet may let you lose about 3 to 5 pounds per week, for an average total weight loss of 44 pounds over 12 weeks.

Losing that amount of weight may improve weight-related medical conditions, including diabetes, high blood pressure, and high cholesterol. But in the long-run, very low-calorie diets aren't more effective than more modest diets. Once you go off a diet, you need to change your lifestyle, committing to healthy eating and regular physical activity.

Are Very Low-Calorie Diets Safe?

Very low-calorie diets are not OK for everyone. Talk to your doctor to see if this kind of diet is appropriate for you.

If your BMI is greater than 30, then very low-calorie diets are generally safe when used under proper medical supervision. For people who are overweight but not obese (BMI of 27-30), very low-calorie diets should be reserved for those who have weight-related medical problems and are under medical supervision.

Very low-calorie-diets are not recommended for pregnant or breastfeeding women, and are not appropriate for children or teens except in specialized treatment programs. They also may not be OK for people over age 50, either, depending on the potential need for medications for pre-existing conditions, as well as the possibility of side effects.

What Are the Side Effects of Very Low-Calorie Diets?

People on a very low-calorie diet for 4 to 16 weeks report minor side effects such as fatigue, constipation, nausea, and diarrhea. These conditions usually improve within a few weeks and rarely prevent people from completing the program.

Gallstones are the most common serious side effect of very low-calorie diets. Gallstones are more common during rapid weight loss. When the body experiences a calorie deficit, it starts to break down fat for energy. The liver then secretes more cholesterol and when combined with bile, can form gallstones.

What Are the Other Drawbacks of Very Low-Calorie Diets?

To be healthy, you need a balance of foods from different food groups. It's difficult to get good nutrition and feel satisfied on a very low-calorie diet. In addition, consuming as few as 800 calories daily may not give you the energy you need for daily living and regular physical activity, especially if you eat the same foods every day.

Talk to your doctor or dietitian to make sure you get the nutrients you need while on a very low-calorie diet.

Very Low-Calorie Diets: What You Need to Know

When you're on a low-calorie diet, you usually get between 800 and 1,500 calories a day. For some people, an alternative for short-term weight loss is a very low-calorie diet.

Many very low-calorie diets are commercially-made formulas of 800 calories or fewer that replace all the food you usually eat. Others, such as the well-known grapefruit diet rely on eating a lot of the same low-calorie food or foods.

Very low-calorie diets are not the same as over-the-counter meal replacements, which you substitute for one or two meals a day.

How Effective Are Very Low-Calorie Diets?

If you have a BMI over 30 (which your doctor will call "obese"), then a very low-calorie diet may let you lose about 3 to 5 pounds per week, for an average total weight loss of 44 pounds over 12 weeks.

Losing that amount of weight may improve weight-related medical conditions, including diabetes, high blood pressure, and high cholesterol. But in the long-run, very low-calorie diets aren't more effective than more modest diets. Once you go off a diet, you need to change your lifestyle, committing to healthy eating and regular physical activity.

Are Very Low-Calorie Diets Safe?

Very low-calorie diets are not OK for everyone. Talk to your doctor to see if this kind of diet is appropriate for you.

If your BMI is greater than 30, then very low-calorie diets are generally safe when used under proper medical supervision. For people who are overweight but not obese (BMI of 27-30), very low-calorie diets should be reserved for those who have weight-related medical problems and are under medical supervision.

Very low-calorie-diets are not recommended for pregnant or breastfeeding women, and are not appropriate for children or teens except in specialized treatment programs. They also may not be OK for people over age 50, either, depending on the potential need for medications for pre-existing conditions, as well as the possibility of side effects.

What Are the Side Effects of Very Low-Calorie Diets?

People on a very low-calorie diet for 4 to 16 weeks report minor side effects such as fatigue, constipation, nausea, and diarrhea. These conditions usually improve within a few weeks and rarely prevent people from completing the program.

Gallstones are the most common serious side effect of very low-calorie diets. Gallstones are more common during rapid weight loss. When the body experiences a calorie deficit, it starts to break down fat for energy. The liver then secretes more cholesterol and when combined with bile, can form gallstones.

What Are the Other Drawbacks of Very Low-Calorie Diets?

To be healthy, you need a balance of foods from different food groups. It's difficult to get good nutrition and feel satisfied on a very low-calorie diet. In addition, consuming as few as 800 calories daily may not give you the energy you need for daily living and regular physical activity, especially if you eat the same foods every day.

Talk to your doctor or dietitian to make sure you get the nutrients you need while on a very low-calorie diet.

The Fast 800 Calorie Diet explained with recipes for breakfast, lunch and dinner

The Fast 800 diet has quickly become one of the most popular weight loss plans out there and has swept the headlines over the last few years, following the widespread success of the 5:2 diet and intermittent fasting.

According to founder Dr Michael Mosley, those who closely follow the plan could see themselves lose up to 11lb in two weeks by limiting their daily intake to 800 calories a day.

It's been praised, alongside the 16:8 diet, as one of the quickest ways to start weight loss through dedicated fasting. Some people also take on the diet because they can't lose weight in other ways and have found fasting to be most effective. But while some health professionals have branded the diet as quick fix and not a long-term way to lose weight healthily, others have said that dieters are eating filling and nutritious foods on the fasting days so it's a relatively healthy way to lose weight, despite the low-calorie intake.

Fans of the diet have also said it does amazing things for your overall health. As well as the physical appearance that many people aspire to have, they claim that the diet also gives your brain a boost, improves your mood and increases your motivation. While some health professionals argue that intermittent fasting diets this this one have the potential to reverse conditions like diabetes and high blood pressure.

As one Twitter user credited founder of the diet, Dr Michael Mosley, 'Lost a stone in 4 weeks & feeling amazing. My hot flushes have reduced, I've got loads of energy & I'm really enjoying life & enjoying cooking. The recipes are delicious!! Thank you to you & your wife for transforming my life for the better..x'

While another wrote, '3 weeks in and lost 12 pounds and 5 inches off my weight – thank you! 👏 👏'

Dr Michael Mosley says himself, "Eating well doesn't just help you lose weight. Good food can boost your immune system, give you energy and even impact your mood.

"It can be pretty confusing to know what we should eat to stay healthy. My advice? Turn to the Med."

This is one of the foundations of the Fast 800 Calorie Diet. Read on to find out more...

What is the Fast 800 Calorie Diet?

The Fast 800 diet involves cutting your calories intake to 800 a day for the first couple of weeks. You then progress to 5:2 stage – where you're only required to eat this number of calories for two days a week, while following a sensible diet on the other days.

Stage 1

Involves sticking to 800 calories a day for at least two weeks. This should induce mild ketosis, associated with fat burning.

Stage 2

The new 5:2. When you're nearing your weight-loss target, eat 800 calories on two days of the week and on the others, follow a Mediterranean diet, exercising portion control.

During this period of the diet, it's advised you enjoy fewer processed and more home-cooked foods, with plenty of vegetables and fruit as well as whole grains, beans, lentils, extra fibre, lots of nuts and plenty of full-fat dairy and oily fish. Sugar should be reduced or avoided, starchy carbs, like white bread and white pasta, are gone, and 45-60g of good-quality protein should be consumed daily.

Why is this stage important? On your two fast days, your body will enter a state of ketosis just as it would if you undertook a rapid weight loss plan. With the new 5:2, you will lose fat and achieve a better response to insulin which will in turn, make it easier for you to keep portion sizes regular during the week.

The new 5:2 also gives those on the plan the chance to experience other fasting benefits, such as apoptosis (clearing out of old or damaged cells), tissue regeneration, reduced risk of cancer, increased metabolic rate and decreased inflammation.

Dr Mosley says, "The Mediterranean diet is the healthiest diet on the planet. There is this perception that Italian food is predominantly pasta and pizza, but this is not true. It's actually packed with fruit, vegetables, nuts, olive oil and fish – all of which are good for you and have been proven to help prevent dementia, strokes, cardiovascular disease, heart disease and has even in some cases, been known to reverse type 2 diabetes."

The main components of the Mediterranean Diet are...

• Daily consumption of vegetables, fruits, whole grains and healthy fats.

• Weekly intake of fish, poultry, beans and eggs.

• Moderate portions of dairy products.

• Limited intake of red meat.

By following the Mediterranean Diet at this stage of the Fast800, you can keep on track and stay healthy.

Stage 3

You've hit your goal, so maintenance is key. Continue the Med-style approach, throwing in the odd fast day as and when, eating a low-sugar diet and moderately low amounts of starchy carbs.

800 calorie meal plan

Below you will find everything you need for an 800 calorie meal plan when you're on the diet. Below are our favourite recipes for breakfast, lunch and dinner for the Fast 800 diet. Who said dieting doesn't mean eating delicious food?

Fast 800 Calorie Diet recipes

The recipes below are all fasting ones, but follow the suggested changes to make them into meals suitable for non-fasting days.

These are featured in The Fast 800 Recipe Book, written by Dr Clare Bailey and Justine Pattison, which is a fabulous companion cookbook to Michael Mosley's bestselling The Fast 800. The recipe book includes more than 130 delicious, low-carb, Mediterranean-style recipes offering multiple options for both 800-calorie days and the new 5:2.

Fast 800 Calorie Diet recipes for breakfast

Spiced breakfast plums (233 cals, serves 2)

1. Put 4 plums, halved and stoned, in a saucepan. Add 2x 10-12cm orange zest strips and 100ml fresh orange juice, 150ml water and ¼tsp ground cinnamon. Stir gently.

2. Bring liquid to a simmer, cover with a lid, reduce the heat to low and cook for 10-15 mins.

3. Divide the spiced plums between two bowls, along with 100g full-fat Greek yogurt and 15g toasted flaked almonds. This can be served warm or cold.

NOT FASTING? Add extra toasted flaked almonds.

TOP TIP: This dish works as a dessert too!

Pear and cinnamon porridge (267 cals, serves 1)

1. Place 30g jumbo oats, ½ pear, cored and chopped, and ¼tsp ground cinnamon into a small non-stick saucepan. Pour in 75ml full-fat milk and 120ml water and cook over a low-medium heat for 5-6 mins, stirring constantly.

2. Pour into a deep bowl and scatter with 5g flaked almonds to serve.

NOT FASTING? Increase the portion size

Poached eggs with mushrooms and spinach (241 cals, serves 1)

1. Third-fill a saucepan with water and bring to a gentle simmer.

2. Break 2 medium eggs into a cup, then carefully tip one at a time into pan. Cook over a very low

heat, with the water hardly bubbling, for 3 mins, or until the whites are set but the yolks remain runny.

3. While poaching the eggs, melt 5g butter in a medium non-stick frying pan over a medium heat and stir-fry 75g small chestnut mushrooms for 2-3 mins.

4. Add 50g spinach and toss with the mushrooms until just wilted. Season with a pinch of sea salt and black pepper.

5. Serve the mushrooms and spinach on plate. Drain the eggs with a slotted spoon and place on top. Serve with more ground black pepper.

NOT FASTING? Serve on top of a slice of wholegrain toast.

Other options include avocado, ricotta and mushrooms (with or without toast) – delicious!

Fast 800 Calorie Diet recipes for lunch

Curried chicken and lentil soup (223 cals, serves 4)

1. Heat 1tbsp extra virgin olive oil in a large non-stick saucepan, add 1 onion, peeled and finely chopped, and 1 pepper, deseeded and cut into chunks, and gently fry for 5 mins. Stir in 2tbsp curry powder and cook for a few seconds more, stirring constantly.

2. Add 1 x 400g can chopped tomatoes and bring to the boil. Cook for 2 mins, stirring constantly,

then crumble over 1 chicken stock cube and add 1 litre water.

3. Rinse 50g dried red split lentils and add to the pan. Stir in 225g frozen spinach and bring to simmer. Season well with salt and pepper. Cook 10 mins, stirring often.

4. Add 200g cooked chicken pieces and cook for 8-10 mins. You can add extra water if needed.

5. Adjust seasoning to taste and serve with lemon wedges for squeezing over.

NOT FASTING? Top with 2tbsp of toasted flaked almonds and 1tbspof full-fat Greek yogurt.

Edamame and tuna salad (408 cals, serves 2)

1. Tip 200g frozen edamame beans into a heatproof bowl and cover with just-boiled water

from a kettle. Stir and leave for 1 min to allow the beans to thaw. Drain and rinse under cold water.

2. Place the beans, 2 spring onions, trimmed and thinly sliced, 1 x 110g no-drain tinned tuna and 15g parsley in a bowl and use a fork to flake the tuna. Drizzle 1½tbsp cider vinegar and 3tbsp olive oil over salad, season with salt and pepper and toss together well.

3. Just before serving, add 2 large handfuls of rocket and toss lightly.

NOT FASTING? Increase the portion size.

Asparagus, pea and mint frittata muffins (154 cals per muffin, serves 6)

1. Preheat the oven to 200C/fan 180C/Gas 6 and generously oil a deep, six-hole muffin tin. Cut six roughly 10cm square pieces of non-stick baking paper and use to line the tins, leaving the excess paper peeking over the sides.

2. Third-fill a large pan with water and bring to the boil. Add 150g asparagus, trimmed and cut into 2-3cm pieces, and cook for 4 mins. Add 100g frozen peas and cook for 1 min more. Drain the vegetables and tip into a large bowl with 4 spring onions, trimmed and thinly sliced, and 3-4tbsp chopped fresh mint.

3. Beat 6 large eggs in a separate bowl with a good pinch of salt and pepper.

4. Divide the vegetables between six muffin cases and top with 65g feta chunks.

5. Pour the egg over the vegetables, then bake in the oven for about 20 mins.

NOT FASTING? Increase the portion size.

Speedy pizza

221 cals I Serves 2

1. Preheat grill to medium-hot setting. For the pizza topping, tip ½ a 400g can of chopped tomatoes into a sieve and shake to remove any excess juice.

2. Transfer the tomato pulp to bowl and stir in 1tbsp tomato purée and ½tsp dried oregano. Season with salt and pepper.

3. Lightly toast 1 wholemeal pitta bread, place on a board and carefully cut in half horizontally with

a bread knife. Separate the two pieces, place on a baking tray, cut side down.

4. Spread the pitta halves with tomato sauce and top with 2 roasted red peppers from a jar, drained and sliced, and 2 chestnut mushrooms, very finely sliced. Sprinkle with 35g grated mozzarella, drizzle with 1tbsp olive oil and place under the grill for 4-5 mins.

We also love this recipe for mushroom stroganoff!

Fast 800 Calorie Diet recipes for dinner

Sausages with onion gravy and cauliflower mash (367 cals, serves 4)

1. For the cauliflower mash, half-fill a medium pan with water and bring to the boil. Add 1 medium

cauliflower, trimmed and cut into small florets and return to the boil. Cook for 15-20 mins or until soft. Drain, then return to the pan. Add 1tbsp olive oil, a couple of pinches of salt and lots of ground black pepper. Blitz in a food processor until smooth. Keep warm over a very low heat, stirring occasionally.

2. Meanwhile, heat 2tbsp olive oil in a large non-stick frying pan and gently fry 12 chipolata sausages for 5 mins, turning regularly. Add 1 onion, peeled and thinly sliced, and cook for a further 8-10 mins.

3. Stir in 300ml hot chicken or pork stock and 2tbsp reduced-sugar tomato ketchup and bring to simmer. Mix 2tsp cornflour with 1tbsp cold water in a small bowl and stir into the pan. Season with

pepper and simmer for 1-2 mins. Adjust the seasoning to taste.

4. Divide the cauliflower mash between four warmed plates and top with the sausages and gravy.

NOT FASTING? Increase the portion size and add a generous knob of butter or grated Cheddar to the cauliflower after blending, and mix thoroughly.

Spicy bean chilli (346 cals, serves 4)

1. Heat 2tbsp oil in a large, deep, non-stick frying pan, and gently fry 1 peeled and sliced onion for 3-4 mins.

2. Add 1tsp smoked paprika, 1tsp cumin and 1tsp ground coriander and cook for a few seconds, stirring well.

3. Add 1 x 400g can of chopped tomatoes, 1 x 400g can of drained black beans and 1 x 400g can of drained mixed beans, 250ml vegetable stock, 1tbsp tomato purée and 1tsp mixed dried herbs, season with salt and pepper and bring to simmer. Cover loosely with lid and cook for 15-20 mins, stirring occasionally.

4. Serve topped with a sprinkling of Cheddar (75g in total) and generous spoonfuls of full-fat Greek yogurt.

NOT FASTING? Serve with cooked brown rice and top with sliced avocado.

Fast 800 Calorie Diet snack recipe

Almond and raisin chocolate pennies (38 cals per penny, makes 20)

1. Line a baking tray with non-stick baking paper.

2. Break 100g plain dark chocolate into squares and place in a bowl over a pan of gently simmering water. Make sure the base of the bowl isn't touching the water. Leave to melt for 5 mins, stirring occasionally. Or, melt in a microwave on high for 1-2 mins.

3. Carefully remove the hot bowl from the pan and, using a teaspoon, pour individual spoonfuls of melted chocolate onto the tray, spaced well apart.

4. Scatter 25g flaked almonds and 25g raisins on top of the melted chocolate. Leave to set for 2-3 hours.

Healthy Eating — A Detailed Guide for Beginners

Why Should You Eat Healthy?

Research continues to link serious diseases to a poor diet.

For example, eating healthy can drastically reduce your chances of developing heart disease and cancer, the world's leading killers.

A good diet can improve all aspects of life, from brain function to physical performance. In fact, food affects all your cells and organs.

If you participate in exercise or sports, there is no doubt that a healthy diet will help you perform better.

Bottom Line:

From disease risk to brain function and physical performance, a healthy diet is vital for every aspect of life.

Calories and Energy Balance Explained

In recent years, the importance of calories has been pushed aside.

While calorie counting isn't always necessary, total calorie intake still plays a key role in weight control and health.

If you put in more calories than you burn, you will store them as new muscle or body fat. If you consume fewer calories than you burn every day, you will lose weight.

If you want to lose weight, you must create some form of calorie deficit

In contrast, if you are trying to gain weight and increase muscle mass, then you need to eat more than your body burns.

Bottom Line:

Calories and energy balance are important, regardless of the composition of your diet.

Understanding Macronutrients

The three macronutrients are carbohydrates (carbs), fats and protein.

These nutrients are needed in relatively large amounts. They provide calories and have various functions in your body.

Here are some common foods within each macronutrient group:

Carbs: 4 calories per gram. All starchy foods like bread, pasta and potatoes. Also includes fruit, legumes, juice, sugar and some dairy products.

Protein: 4 calories per gram. Main sources include meat and fish, dairy, eggs, legumes and vegetarian alternatives like tofu.

Fats: 9 calories per gram. Main sources include nuts, seeds, oils, butter, cheese, oily fish and fatty meat.

How much of each macronutrient you should consume depends on your lifestyle and goals, as well as your personal preferences.

Bottom Line:

Macronutrients are the three main nutrients needed in large amounts: carbs, fats and protein.

Understanding Micronutrients

Micronutrients are important vitamins and minerals that you require in smaller doses.

Some of the most common micronutrients you should know include:

Magnesium: Plays a role in over 600 cellular processes, including energy production, nervous system function and muscle contraction.

Potassium: This mineral is important for blood pressure control, fluid balance and the function of your muscles and nerves.

Iron: Primarily known for carrying oxygen in the blood, iron also has many other benefits, including improved immune and brain function.

Calcium: An important structural component of bones and teeth, and also a key mineral for your heart, muscles and nervous system.

All vitamins: The vitamins, from vitamin A to K, play important roles in every organ and cell in your body.

All of the vitamins and minerals are "essential" nutrients, meaning that you must get them from the diet in order to survive.

The daily requirement of each micronutrient varies between individuals. If you eat a real food-based diet that includes plants and animals, then you should get all the micronutrients your body needs without taking a supplement.

Bottom Line:

Micronutrients are important vitamins and minerals that play key roles in your cells and organs.

Eating Whole Foods is Important

You should aim to consume whole foods at least 80-90% of the time.

The term "whole foods" generally describes natural, unprocessed foods containing only one ingredient.

If the product looks like it was made in a factory, then it's probably not a whole food.

Whole foods tend to be nutrient-dense and have a lower energy density. This means that they have fewer calories and more nutrients per serving than processed foods.

In contrast, many processed foods have little nutritional value and are often referred to as "empty" calories. Eating them in large amounts is linked to obesity and other diseases.

Bottom Line:

Basing your diet on whole foods is an extremely effective but simple strategy to improve health and lose weight.

Foods to Eat

Try to base your diet around these healthy food groups:

Vegetables: These should play a fundamental role at most meals. They are low in calories yet full of important micronutrients and fiber.

Fruits: A natural sweet treat, fruit provides micronutrients and antioxidants that can help improve health.

Meat and fish: Meat and fish have been the major sources of protein throughout evolution. They are a staple in the human diet, although vegetarian and vegan diets have become popular as well.

Nuts and seeds: These are one of the best fat sources available and also contain important micronutrients.

Eggs: Considered one of the healthiest foods on the planet, whole eggs pack a powerful combination of protein, beneficial fats and micronutrients.

Dairy: Dairy products such as natural yogurt and milk are convenient, low-cost sources of protein and calcium.

Healthy starches: For those who aren't on a low-carb diet, whole food starchy foods like potatoes, quinoa and Ezekiel bread are healthy and nutritious.

Beans and legumes: These are fantastic sources of fiber, protein and micronutrients.

Beverages: Water should make up the majority of your fluid intake, along with drinks like coffee and tea.

Herbs and spices: These are often very high in nutrients and beneficial plant compounds.

For a longer list, here is an article with 50 super healthy foods.

Bottom Line:

Base your diet on these healthy whole foods and ingredients. They will provide all the nutrients your body needs.

Weight management options have evolved

Take our quiz to learn more about techniques and tips that will help you achieve your goals.

Foods to Avoid Most of the Time

By following the advice in this article, you will naturally reduce your intake of unhealthy foods.

No food needs to be eliminated forever, but some foods should be limited or saved for special occasions.

These include:

Sugar-based products: Foods high in sugar, especially sugary drinks, are linked to obesity and type 2 diabetes.

Trans fats: Also known as partially hydrogenated fats, trans fats have been linked to serious diseases, such as heart disease.

Refined carbs: Foods that are high in refined carbs, such as white bread, are linked to overeating, obesity and metabolic disease).

Vegetable oils: While many people believe these are healthy, vegetable oils can disrupt your body's omega 6-to-3 balance, which may cause problems.

Processed low-fat products: Often disguised as healthy alternatives, low-fat products usually contain a lot of sugar to make them taste better.

Bottom Line:

While no food is strictly off limits, overeating certain foods can increase disease risk and lead to weight gain.

Why Portion Control is Important

Your calorie intake is a key factor in weight control and health.

By controlling your portions, you are more likely to avoid consuming too many calories.

While whole foods are certainly a lot harder to overeat than processed foods, they can still be eaten in excess.

If you are overweight or trying to lose body fat, it's particularly important to monitor your portion size.

There are many simple strategies to control portion size.

For example, you can use smaller plates and take a smaller-than-average first serving, then wait 20 minutes before you return for more.

Another popular approach is measuring portion size with your hand. An example meal would limit most people to 1 fist-sized portion of carbs, 1–2 palms of protein and 1–2 thumb-sized portions of healthy fats.

More calorie-dense foods such as cheese, nuts and fatty meats are healthy, but make sure you pay attention to portion sizes when you eat them.

Bottom Line:

Be aware of portion sizes and your total food or calorie intake, especially if you are overweight or trying to lose fat.

How to Tailor Your Diet to Your Goals

First, assess your calorie needs based on factors like your activity levels and weight goals.

Quite simply, if you want to lose weight, you must eat less than you burn. If you want to gain weight, you should consume more calories than you burn.

Here is a calorie calculator that tells you how much you should eat, and here are 5 free websites and apps that help you track calories and nutrients.

If you dislike calorie counting, you can simply apply the rules discussed above, such as monitoring portion size and focusing on whole foods.

If you have a certain deficiency or are at risk of developing one, you may wish to tailor your diet to account for this. For instance, vegetarians or people who eliminate certain food groups are at greater risk of missing out on some nutrients.

In general, you should consume foods of various types and colors to ensure you get plenty of all the macro- and micronutrients.

While many debate whether low-carb or low-fat diets are best, the truth is that it depends on the individual.

Based on research, athletes and those looking to lose weight should consider increasing their protein intake. In addition, a lower-carb diet may work wonders for some individuals trying to lose weight or treat type 2 diabetes.

Bottom Line:

Consider your total calorie intake and adjust your diet based on your own needs and goals.

How to Make Healthy Eating Sustainable

Here's a great rule to live by: If you can't see yourself on this diet in one, two or three years, then it's not right for you.

Far too often, people go on extreme diets they can't maintain, which means they never actually develop long-term, healthy eating habits.

There are some frightening weight gain statistics showing that most people regain all the weight they lost soon after attempting a weight loss diet.

As always, balance is key. Unless you have a specific disease or dietary requirement, no food needs to be off limits forever. By totally eliminating certain foods, you may actually increase cravings and decrease long-term success.

Basing 90% of your diet on whole foods and eating smaller portions will allow you to enjoy treats occasionally yet still achieve excellent health.

This is a far healthier approach than doing the opposite and eating 90% processed food and only 10% whole food like many people do.

Bottom Line:

Create a healthy diet that you can enjoy and stick with for the long term. If you want unhealthy foods, save them for an occasional treat.

Consider These Supplements

As the name suggests, supplements are meant to be used in addition to a healthy diet.

Including plenty of nutrient-dense foods in your diet should help you reverse deficiencies and meet all your daily needs.

However, a few well-researched supplements have been shown to be helpful in some cases.

One example is vitamin D, which is naturally obtained from sunlight and foods like oily fish. Most people have low levels or are deficient.

Supplements like magnesium, zinc and omega-3s can provide additional benefits if you do not get enough of them from your diet.

Other supplements can be used to enhance sports performance. Creatine, whey protein and beta-alanine all have plenty of research supporting their use.

In a perfect world, your diet would be full of nutrient-dense foods with no need for supplements. However, this isn't always achievable in the real world.

If you are already making a constant effort to improve your diet, additional supplements can help take your health a step further.

Bottom Line:

It is best to get most of your nutrients from whole foods. However, some supplements can be useful as well.

Combine Good Nutrition With Other Healthy Habits

Nutrition isn't the only thing that matters for optimal health.

Following a healthy diet and exercising can give you an even bigger health boost.

It is also crucial to get good sleep. Research shows that sleep is just as important as nutrition for disease risk and weight control.

Hydration and water intake are also important. Drink when you're thirsty and stay well hydrated all day.

Finally, try to minimize stress. Long-term stress is linked to many health problems.

Bottom Line:

Optimal health goes way beyond just nutrition. Exercising, getting good sleep and minimizing stress is also crucial.

Take Home Message

The strategies outlined above will drastically improve your diet.

They will also boost your health, lower your disease risk and help you lose weight.

www.ingramcontent.com/pod-product-compliance
Lightning Source LLC
Chambersburg PA
CBHW071024260726
48662CB00024B/1936